Sarah Ingrid Pinto Santos
Amanda Taylla Lima Silva
Alessandra Lima Rocha

Influence of the use of contraceptive drugs

Sarah Ingrid Pinto Santos
Amanda Taylla Lima Silva
Alessandra Lima Rocha

Influence of the use of contraceptive drugs

In the Development of Pyometra

ScienciaScripts

Imprint

Cover image: www.ingimage.com

This book is a translation from the original published under ISBN 978-613-9-61342-7.

Publisher:
Sciencia Scripts
is a trademark of
Dodo Books Indian Ocean Ltd. and OmniScriptum S.R.L publishing group

120 High Road, East Finchley, London, N2 9ED, United Kingdom
Str. Armeneasca 28/1, office 1, Chisinau MD-2012, Republic of Moldova, Europe
Printed at: see last page
ISBN: 978-620-8-16688-5

"First of all, the most important thing is that you want to care for all kinds of animals and really want to improve their health and well being - this is why we become vets and vet nurses after all."

(Noel Fitzpatrick)

I dedicate this work to my grandparents Firmino Teixeira Santos and Rosimar Pinto Santos *(in memoriam)* with all my love and gratitude, for everything they have done for me throughout my life. I wish I could have been worthy of the effort you dedicated to me in every way, especially with regard to my education.

(Sarah Ingrid Pinto Santos)

SUMMARY

Reproductive control in pets is a very pertinent issue for owners who can opt for the surgical sterilisation method or the use of reversible contraceptive drugs. Although the surgical method is more effective and safer, many owners find it costly and adopt contraceptive drugs. However, the use of these drugs can lead to a series of pathologies, including pyometra, dead foetuses and mammary tumours. As a result, this study aimed to assess cases of pyometra, relating them to age, race and contraceptive use. The clinical records of 2,325 females treated at the HVU - UEMA in 2016 were analysed and 271 of these were diagnosed with pathologies associated with the use of contraceptives. Of these, 112 were positive for pyomctra. Adult female dogs aged between 3 and 6 years were predisposed to developing pyometra. There was no racial predisposition to the condition, as in other similar studies. The use of contraceptives in bitches with pyometra corresponded to a large part of the data collected, showing an alarming situation. It is therefore possible to state that there was indiscriminate use of contraceptives by owners, which led to the development of the pathology studied. It is therefore essential that owners are made aware of the risks these drugs pose to the health and well-being of female dogs and are informed about the safety and efficacy of the surgical sterilisation method.

Keywords: contraceptives; pyometra; dogs.

SUMMARY

CHAPTER 1

INTRODUCTION

The domestication of dogs and cats, which dates back more than ten thousand years, has been present since the development of human relationships based on group dynamics and was a process intrinsic to urbanisation, which made these animals revered as family members (BECK, 1973). This relationship intensified from the 16th and 17th centuries onwards, when the improvement in man's quality of life allowed animals to be bred without an economic function, just for companionship (THOMAS, 1988).

Since then, the pet population has grown significantly, reaching around 1.51 billion worldwide and 74.2 million in Brazil (IBGE, 2015). However, the high growth in the population of these animals associated with uncontrolled breeding and irresponsible owners has led to the proliferation of stray dogs and cats in large urban centres, giving rise to overpopulation and its consequences for public health (LIMA E LUNA, 2012).

The main problems arising from living with stray animals in urban areas are car accidents, damage to the environment, the spread of infectious and parasitic diseases (zoonoses) and bites (SINAN, 2009).

For reproductive control, owners can opt for the surgical sterilisation method or the use of reversible contraceptive drugs. The surgical method is more effective and safer, while the use of drugs exposes females to a series of risks (NEVES et al., 2003).

Some owners consider the surgical sterilisation method to be costly and therefore adopt pharmacological contraception as a low-cost alternative, easily found in farm shops and sold without a veterinary prescription (OLIVEIRA E MARQUES JÚNIOR, 2006).

However, the use of contraceptives in domestic animals can cause a series of reproductive problems, favouring the occurrence of mammary or uterine neoplasms, cystic endometrial hyperplasia with subsequent uterine infection (pyometra) and, if applied to pregnant women, can cause delayed delivery, dystocia and retained foetuses, foetal maceration and abortion (DE NARDI et al., 2002; FILGUEIRA et al., 2008; BACARDO et al., 2008; ARAÚJO, 2013).

The aim of this study was to analyse the cases of pyometra in female dogs treated with contraceptive drugs at the Veterinary Hospital of the State University of Maranhão in 2016.

CHAPTER 2

LITERATURE REVIEW

2.1. ANATOMY OF THE REPRODUCTIVE SYSTEM FEMALE

The reproductive system of bitches is made up of the ovaries, fallopian tubes, uterus, vagina, vestibule and vulva, as shown in **Figure 1**. All these structures play a fundamental role in providing conception, pregnancy and delivery of viable offspring (FOSTER, 2009).

The structures of the female reproductive tract are analogous to the male genital organs and are divided into gamete-producing structures and those responsible for transporting and storing the gametes formed **(Konig & Liebich, 2016)**.

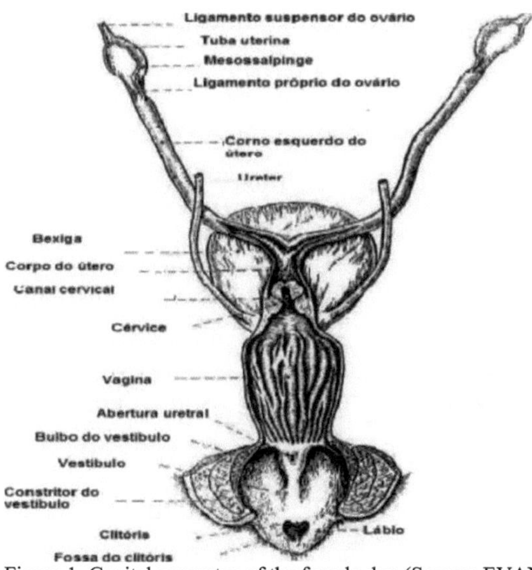

Figure 1. Genital apparatus of the female dog (Source: EVANS and DELAHUNTA, 2001).

1.1.2. Ovaries

A small number of primordial germ cells migrate from the yolk sac to the gonadal primordia in the first month of embryonic life. In these gonads, which are beginning to develop, the cells divide to form ovogonia (Junqueira & Carneiro, 2013).

In the third month of gestation, the first meiotic division of the ovogonia begins, with a pause in division in the diplotene phase. These cells are called primary oocytes and are only released by the oocytes at puberty in females (Junqueira & Carneiro, 2013).

The main functions of the ovaries are oogenesis and steroidogenesis of oestrogen and progesterone (DUKES, 1996). They are arranged in pairs and have an oval shape, an elongated and flattened outline, measuring around 2 cm in diameter, but their dimensions can change according to the phase of the oestrus cycle.

They are located between 1 and 2 cm caudal to the kidney on the corresponding side, attached to the dorsolateral region of the abdominal wall via the broad ligament of the uterus (GETTY, 1986; FELDMAN and NELSON, 2003). The right ovary is positioned more cranially than the left, dorsal to the descending duodenum, while the left ovary is dorsal to the descending colon and lateral to the spleen (FOSSUM, 2008).

The ovaries of bitches are surrounded by the ovarian sac, a structure completely covered by adipose tissue from the mesovarium and mesosalpinx (SLATTER, 2007). The ovarian arteries are responsible for the blood supply to the ovaries and arise from the abdominal aorta in the left ovary and the renal artery in the right ovary (FINGLAND, 1996).

In a longitudinal section, you can see a vascular zone in the centre, the medulla, and a surrounding layer, the parenchymatous zone. This zone is reversed by the tunica albuginea. The medulla of the ovary is made up of vessels, nerves, lymphatics, muscle fibres and connective tissue, while the parenchymatous zone has several follicles and corpora lutea (**KONIG and LIEBITH, 2016**).

Ovarian follicles are formed in the parenchymal zone of the ovaries. Follicles are responsible for the entire process of oogenesis, behaving like an endocrine gland that produces steroids and releases oocytes (KONIG and LIEBITH, 2016; EPPIG, 2001).

1.1.3. Uterine tube

The fallopian tubes are small sinuous structures between 5 and 9 cm long. They originate on the medial surface of the ovaries and have the function of receiving and conducting the oocytes released by the ovaries during ovulation and providing fertilisation by sperm (SLATTER, 2007).

They have three well-defined segments surrounded by the mesosalpinx, these being the infundibulum, which has fimbriae partially attached to the respective ovary, helping to capture the oocytes, the ampulla which is a wider region where fertilisation takes place and the isthmus which is where the fallopian tube attaches to the uterus (KONIG and LIEBICH, 2004; FEITOSA, 2014).

The mesovarium and mesosalpinx act as suspensors for the ovaries and fallopian tubes and are known as the broad ligament of the uterus. Nerves and blood vessels pass through this ligament, feeding these organs. In addition to the mesovarium, bitches have their own ovarian ligament. In bitches, the mesovarium, mesosalpinx and ligamentum propria form the ovarian sac that surrounds the entire ovary (KONIG and LIEBITCH, 2004).

1.1.4. Uterus

The uterus is the hollow muscular organ that houses the foetus during pregnancy and is made up of the cervix, the body and two uterine horns (COLVILLE, 2010). The cervix is the region corresponding to the entrance to the uterus and is thicker than the other adjacent structures, remaining closed for most of the oestrus cycle, preserving the uterus' sterility (FELDMAN and NELSON, 2003). The body is shorter than the uterine horns, approximately 1.5 cm long, and acts to direct the foetuses towards the cervix at the time of parturition (GETTY, 1986; SLATTER, 2007). The uterine horns are more elongated than the other regions of the uterus and are connected cranially to the fallopian tubes and caudally to the uterine body. It is the place where pregnancy develops (FELDMAN and NELSON, 2003).

The uterus has three distinct layers that are internal, intermediate and external: the endometrium, myometrium and perimetrium, respectively (JOHSNTON, 2001). The endometrium is endowed with secretory functions of mucus and other substances from the simple columnar epithelium and tubular glands that line it. The myometrium is the muscular layer formed by smooth muscle that acts during labour to expel the offspring into the external environment. The perimetrium is closely linked to the myometrial musculature and is the outermost layer of the uterus, lined by the peritoneum (COLVILLE, 2010).

The ovarian and uterine arteries are responsible for the blood supply to the uterus. While only the cranial portion of the uterine horn is irrigated by the ovarian artery, most of the uterus, corresponding to the caudal portion, is irrigated by the uterine artery (SLATTER, 2007).

1.1.5. Vagina

The vagina is moderately long and cranially narrow, with longitudinal muscular folds responsible for its distension capacity. It is located ventrally to the lower urinary tract and dorsally to the rectum. This structure extends from the external uterine ostium to the external ostium of the urethra (DYCE, SACK and WENSING, 1997; GETTY, 1989; KONIG and LIEBITH, 2004).

The vaginal vestibule combines reproductive and urinary functions. It is largely located behind the ischial arch and its wall has vestibular glands, whose function is to keep the vestibular mucosa moist, facilitating coitus and labour (KONIG and LIEBITH, 2004).

1.1.6. Ligaments

Double folds of peritoneum form the broad ligaments of the uterus (right and left), considered the main attachment of this organ. These ligaments suspend the ovaries, fallopian tubes and uterus from the abdominal and pelvic walls (KONIG and LIEBITH, 2004).

The broad ligaments are divided into the mesovarium, which holds the ovary; the mesosalpinx, the oviduct and the mesometrium, which anchors the uterus. The mesovarium is made up of the ovarian artery and vein. The serous membranes of the ligament are separated by smooth muscle from the myometrium (KONIG and LIEBITH, 2004; FEITOSA, 2014).

In addition to the broad ligaments, there is also the round ligament of the uterus in the female reproductive system. This is a cord of fibrous tissue and smooth muscle, located at the free edge of the lateral fold of the broad ligament. It extends from the caudal region of the uterine horn to the ventral area of the inguinal ring (COLVILLE, 2010).

1.1.7. Vulva

The vulva is the external portion of the reproductive tract, easily visible without the need for handling and located in the caudal terminal portion of the vestibule (JOHNSTON, 2001). It has a pair of labia and the external urogenital orifice, which make up the labial commissure directed in a dorso-ventral direction (EVANS and DELAHUNTA, 2001). Depending on the phase of the oestrus cycle, bitches may have a moderately small or very swollen vulva, which is an excellent parameter for determining proestrus (CONCANNON, 2005).

1.1.8. Vascularisation

The female reproductive tract is irrigated by four arteries: the ovarian, uterine, vaginal and internal pudendal arteries. The ovarian arteries irrigate the ovary and give off branches to the fallopian tube and uterine horn. The branches that go to the uterus unite with the uterine artery inside the broad ligament (KONIG and LIEBITH, 2004).

According to Konig and Liebith (2004), the ovarian artery originates from the aorta, while the vaginal artery comes from the internal iliac arteries. The uterine artery is a branch of the vaginal artery, which supplies the uterine horns and bodies. The caudal region of the female genital system is irrigated by branches of the pudendal and vaginal arteries.

The ovarian, uterine and vaginal veins are branches of the arteries. The ovarian vein drains most of the uterus and is considered larger than the uterine vein. The vaginal vein drains a large part of the vagina and vestibule (KONIG and LIEBITH, 2004).

1.2. STAR CYCLE

Puberty marks the beginning of sexual activity in bitches, occurring between 6 and 18 months of age. From then on, the hormonal activities characteristic of the oestrus cycle last for 3 months, coinciding at the end with anestrus, the period in which these activities cease and this last phase continues, establishing an interval of 7 months between each cycle (WANKE and GOBELLO, 2006). Thus, the bitch is monoestrous, as she has one to two oestrous periods per year, with the lutein phase being long and indifferent between pregnant and non-pregnant females (CONCANNON et al., 1989). The bitch's oestrus cycle can be divided into four phases: proestrus, oestrus, diestrus and anestrus (JEFFCOATE and LINDSAY, 1989). Proestrus corresponds to the follicular phase, while oestrus and diestrus correspond to the luteal phase and oestrus to the quiescent phase (ETTINGER, 1992).

1.2.2. Proestro

Proestrus lasts an average of 9 days and can vary from 3 to 21 days and is characterised by clinically visible changes such as vulvar oedema and serosanguinous to bloody vaginal discharge (CONCANNON, 2005). In addition to these changes, proestrus is marked by dilation of the cervix, thickening of the endometrium, growth of the mammary glands as well as an increase in their glandular function. Behaviour can also be altered, especially the rejection of the male for copulation, as well as restlessness, disobedience, polyuria and polydpsia (CHRISTIANSEN, 1988). These changes occur due to an increase in serum oestradiol concentrations (FELDMAN and NELSON, 2003).

The morphological and behavioural changes of this phase occur due to the rise in serum oestradiol concentrations. The developing ovarian follicles synthesise oestradiol in response to the action of FSH on them. These serum oestradiol concentrations rise throughout proestrus up to 24 to 48 hours before the pre-ovulatory peak of luteinising hormone (LH) that will trigger ovulation and initiate oestrus (WANKE and GOBELLO, 2006).

1.2.3. Estro

Oestrus lasts an average of 12 days in bitches, but can vary from 4 to 24 days and is characterised by the period of receptivity of the male to the female, allowing coitus (OLSON and NETT, 1986; GUIDO, 2003). This behavioural change is the result of an increase in serum progesterone levels, which begins with a decrease in oestrogen levels 48 hours before the pre-ovulatory LH peak (WEILENMANN et al., 1993).

The pre-ovulatory LH peak marks the beginning of oestrus and after this phenomenon, there is ovulation and changes in the mature follicles, which undergo luteinisation and begin to synthesise progesterone, further increasing their serum levels (ALLEN, 1995; FELDMAN and NELSON, 2003).

Under the effect of the high level of progesterone, bitches show some behaviours typical of oestrus, such as elevation of the pelvic region to show the perineal region and movement of the tail to one side. Morphological changes are also visualised, such as a less swollen vulva, transparent or straw-yellow discharge without the presence of blood and a less swollen endometrium (CHRISTIANSEN, 1988).

According to Holst and Phemister (1975), maximum fertility can be achieved with successful matings between days zero and five of the LH surge. Meanwhile, Feldman and Nelson (2003) deny that pregnancies can be achieved by mating nine to ten days after the LH peak.

The end of oestrus can be recorded by observing the rejection of the male by the female, but vaginal cytology is more accurate (FELDMAN and NELSON, 2003).

1.2.4. Diestro

The diestrus period follows the end of oestrus, lasts 2 to 3 months, has progesterone as its predominant hormone and is characterised by the rejection of the male (HARVEY, 2006).

During diestrus, the serum concentration of progesterone is similar between pregnant and non-pregnant bitches. This is due to the inability of uterine prostaglandins to cause lysis of the corpus luteum (CL). As a result of the physiological similarities, non-pregnant bitches can develop pseudopregnancy syndrome, marked by the development of mammary glands, uterine secretion, nest building, adoption of inanimate objects, among other alterations reminiscent of maternal behaviour (CHRISTANSEN, 1998; FELDMAN and NELSON, 2003).

In the second half of the diestrous period, serum progesterone declines, stimulating the synthesis and secretion of prolactin and LH. Both hormones are responsible for maintaining the LC during this period, since in the first half of diestrus it is believed that the LC has hormone-independent characteristics (HOFFMAN et al., 1992; JOHNSTON et al., 2001).

1.2.5. Anestro

Anestrus is the phase of reproductive quiescence, characterised by sexual inactivity and the absence of any clinical signs. It can last from 1 to 6 months, with an average of 125 days. During this period, the uterus is in the process of involution, recovering from the physiological changes it underwent in the previous cycle and preparing for the next cycle (CONCANNON, 2008).

Hormonal activities involving the pituitary-ovarian axis and the uterus remain active, however, the ovaries show low responsiveness to gonadotrophins due to the effect of prolactin still present in the circulation (JEFFCOATE, 1993).

The end of anestrus is marked by an increase in the concentration of FSH and oestradiol, starting a new cycle (KOOISTRA et al., 1999).

1.3. PHYSIOLOGY OF PREGNANCY

Pregnancy begins with the fertilisation of the oocytes by the sperm, which in bitches takes place in the fallopian tube. The gestation period can be counted from the time of foaling, which is on average 63 days and can vary from 56 to 72 days (LINDE- FORSBERG and ENEROTH, 2000). This long range of variations is due to the longevity of the dog's sperm in the bitch's reproductive system, which can last up to 7 days (CONCANNON et al.,

2001). There are also other factors that can influence the duration of pregnancy, such as litter size, age of the female and breed (EILTS et al., 2005). However, when considering the LH peak as the starting point for establishing gestation length, the variations are minimal, at 65±1 days (CONCANNON et al, 1989).

The embryo formed as a result of fertilisation will go through the cleavage process until it reaches the blastomere form around day 11 and migrates to the uterus for implantation (CONCANNON et al., 1989).

Around the 18th day of gestation, embryos begin to secrete proteins that help in the implantation process (THATCHER et al., 1995). While still in blastocyst form, the embryo also secretes substances responsible for prolonging the life of the corpus luteum, the structure responsible for secreting progesterone and maintaining pregnancy (HAFEZ and HAFEZ, 2004).

From the 22nd day after embryo implantation, the placenta begins to form in the endometrium. The placenta in bitches is of the circular zonaria type, as there are four distinct layers that accommodate the foetus (MIGLINO et al., 2006).

The development of pregnancy basically depends on high serum concentrations of progesterone produced by the corpus luteum, initially formed after ovulation (LUZ et al., 2006). Situations such as hypoluteoidism or luteolysis are inconceivable for maintaining pregnancy, as progesterone levels will be insufficient, resulting in embryonic or foetal death (LUZ et al., 2004).

Progesterone is responsible for developing the endometrium, making it suitable for supporting the embryo, as well as maintaining placental integrity, reducing myometrial activity and making the uterus less sensitive to oxytocin, establishing the ideal uterine environment for a successful pregnancy (CONCANNON et al., 2001).

It is known that serum levels of progesterone, prolactin and oestrogen in pregnant and non-pregnant bitches during metestrus are similar, which is not a good parameter to indicate conception (HAFEZ and HAFEZ, 2004). However, the hormone relaxin is characteristic of pregnancy and can be detected from the 26th to 30th day of gestation (CONCANNON et al., 1996).

At the end of gestation, the foetus-placenta unit will secrete Prostagladin 2 a (PGF2a) in significant quantities to cause luteolysis. The dissolution of CL will result in the suppression of serum progesterone levels and, consequently, myometrial contraction and labour (CONCANNON et al., 2001).

Another event resulting from the final phase of pregnancy is closely related to the function of the mammary glands. The plasma concentration of prolactin is high and reaches its peak at labour, stimulating lactogenesis (GREGERSON, 2006). However, the proliferative changes in mammary tissue that prepare these glands for colostrum production are closely related to the action of progesterone during pregnancy, stimulating the synthesis of growth hormone in the alveolar lobes (BERNSTEDM and ROSS, 1993).

1.4. CONTRACEPTIVE DRUGS USED

In an attempt to control dog reproduction, many owners adopt the use of contraceptive drugs in female dogs. However, this method is often used without individual assessment, especially with regard to the phase of the oestrus cycle they are in, which can lead to a series of complications (CRAIG, 1996).

The main drugs used are synthetic analogues of progesterone, also known as progestogens, which have a similar mechanism of action to the endogenous hormone, but with prolonged activity (FILGUEIRA et al., 2008).

These contraceptives can be found in oral or injectable form. However, injectable administration is the most widely used among guardians because it provides a longer duration of action (VIGO et al., 2011).

Currently, a wide variety of progestogens can be found on the market, including medroxyprogesterone acetate, megestrol acetate, delmadinone acetate, chlormadinone acetate, cyproterone acetate, melengestrol and proligestone (ENGLAND, 1998; MADDISON et al., 2010).

All of these drugs are intended to prevent oestrus, thus avoiding an undesirable pregnancy (LADDS et al., 1994). They act by inhibiting the secretion of the gonadotropins FSH and LH through their negative feedback effect on the hypothalamus, preventing the growth of ovarian follicles and reducing estrogen levels, consequently stopping ovulation and the sexual behaviour linked to it (CHRISTIANSEN, 1988; KATZUNG, 2003; AGUIAR MOREIRA and PORTO, 2016).

It is recommended that the bitch be assessed individually to determine the current phase of the oestrus cycle, thus avoiding the application of the contraceptive in the proestrus, oestrus and metestrus phases (MONTANHA, CORRÊA and PARRA, 2012).

However, a large number of owners do not seek advice from their veterinarian and disregard the instructions on the package leaflet, an attitude that favours the development of various pathologies (LIMA et al., 2009), such as cystic endometrial hyperplasia, pyometra, foetal retention and death, mammary hyperplasia, mammary neoplasms, pseudocyesis, diabetes mellitus and hypoadrenocorticism which, even in therapeutic doses, can lead to the development of the same conditions (SIMPSON et al., 1998).

Many of these pathologies require urgent surgical intervention due to the risk of death. Therefore, surgical sterilisation has been advocated as the ideal method of reproductive control for female dogs, as it offers safety and prevents the development of these diseases (HONORIO et al., 2016).

1.5. REPRODUCTIVE TRACT PATHOLOGIES RELATED TO CONTRACEPTIVE USE

Pathologies of the reproductive system in female dogs are very common in day-to-day veterinary practice. They are influenced by age, reproductive history, environmental conditions and the use of contraceptives (PREVIATO et al., 2005).

Some of these pathologies stand out for their high incidence and varied mortality rates, where treatment in most cases is surgical and fundamental for the recovery of the affected female (STEPHEN and SHERDING, 2008). Thus, pyometra, fetal retention and death and mammary tumours are among the most prevalent pathologies in the reproductive tract and are highly influenced by the use of contraceptives, as proven in a study by Araújo et al. (2016).

1.5.2. Pyometra

Pyometra is an acute and emergency pathology characterised by the accumulation of infectious purulent material inside the uterus that develops from the cystic endometrial hyperplasia (CEH) complex associated with bacterial infection and causes serious complications to the body when not treated in time, such as acute renal failure and sepsis (ARNOLD et al., 2006; FERREIRA, 2006).

HEC, in turn, is characterised by the growth of endometrial glands and an increase in their secretory activity, stimulated by the prolonged activity of endogenous or exogenous progesterone on receptors located in the endometrium. The secretions of these glands accumulate in the uterine lumen, providing the ideal environment for bacterial growth (SUGIURA et al., 2004). In addition, progesterone reduces myometrial contractility and suppresses local leukocyte activity, which contributes to the retention of secretions in the uterine lumen and the establishment of the infectious process (PRETZER, 2008; SMITH, 2006).

Considering the fundamental role of progesterone in the development of ECH, this condition occurs more frequently during diestrus, a phase of the oestrus cycle in which the corpus luteum keeps serum progesterone levels high for a relatively long period, lasting up to 70 days (HARDY and OBSORNE, 1974). After repeated oestrus cycles, these effects of progesterone on the endometrium are cumulative, meaning that adult and older females are more susceptible to developing this pathology (NELSON and COUTO, 2006). However, this disease can occur at any stage of the oestrus cycle and in females of any age, especially when exogenous progesterone is administered (FERREIRA and LOPES, 2000).

Oestrogen also influences the onset of the disease as it increases the number of progesterone receptors in the endometrium, further inciting the appearance of HEC, as well as opening up the cervix so that pathogens can enter the uterine lumen. Therefore, oestrogen-based contraceptives also present a potential risk in the development of pyometra (NELSON and COUTO, 2006).

A study by Pretzer (2008) reports that bacterial contamination of the uterus probably occurs before diestrus, when the cervix is open, and in cases of HEC, the bacteria cannot be eliminated before the luteal phase, allowing opportunistic organisms to remain in an excellent environment for their colonisation and proliferation, thus triggering pyometra.

These bacteria come largely from the vaginal microfauna and reach the uterus by ascending. The main etiological agent is Escherichia coli, but other microorganisms that are also present in the vagina in healthy conditions can ascend and trigger the same pathological process, such as Streptococcus spp., Staphylococcus aureus spp., Proteus spp., Enterococcus spp., Pasteurella spp., Serratia spp., Haemophillus spp. and Bacillus spp. (ANDRADE, 2002; MARTINS, 2007).

Affected females may have vaginal discharge with an odour characteristic of suppuration in the case of open cervix pyometra, or not in the case of closed cervix pyometra. In addition, they may also show abdominal pain and distension, lethargy, apathy, anorexia, polyuria, polydipsia, vomiting, fever, among other characteristic signs of Acute Renal Failure (ARF) or sepsis (HANGMAN et al, 2006).

When the cervix is open and the purulent secretion drains through the vagina, the uterine horns remain slightly dilated, the uterine wall is thickened and the myometrium is hypertrophied. Under these conditions, the onset of septicaemia is lower and the chances of uterine rupture are minimal, which makes the prognosis favourable for affected females. On the other hand, when the cervix is closed, the uterine horns are distended, the uterine wall is thinned and the endometrium is atrophied, with lymphocytic and plasmacytic infiltrates. In these circumstances, the risk is eminent as there is greater absorption of pathogenic microorganisms and a high probability of uterine rupture (SMITH, 2006).

Once pyometra has set in, its resolution is difficult due to the lack of contraction of the myometrium and failure to relax the cervix, even when bitches have baseline plasma progesterone concentrations. Given the severity of this pathology, even in cases of open pyometra, the treatment of choice is emergency ovariosalpingohysterectomy (FELDMAN and NELSON, 2003; VERSTEGEN et al., 2008). Figure 4 concisely illustrates the pathophysiology of pyometra.

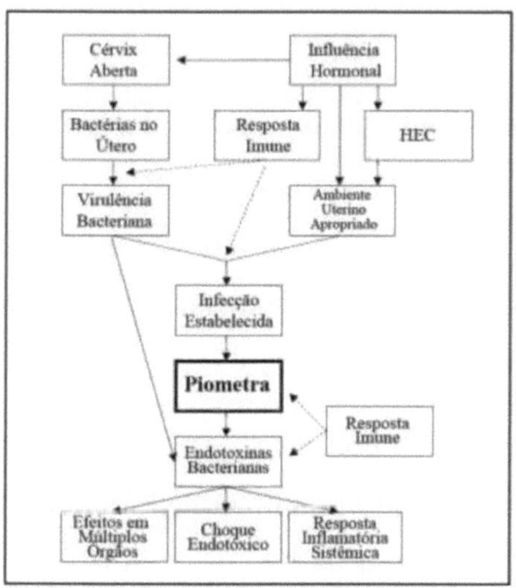

Figure 2: Schematic representation of the pathophysiology of pyometra.
(Source: HAGMAN, 2004).

1.5.3. Foetal retention and death

Foetal death can occur due to various factors related to endocrine, nutritional, traumatic, infectious or congenital alterations in the reproductive tract of the pregnant female (ALVES, 2012). With regard to endocrine factors, the use of contraceptives stands out for causing a disorder in the plasma concentrations of hormones that are fundamental to the continuity of pregnancy, from conception to labour (LUZ et al., 2005).

Under normal conditions, there is a decline in serum P4 levels and an increase in oestrogen in response to the release of foetal cortisol days before parturition, allowing the activity of prostaglandins and oxytocin in uterine contraction. However, when contraceptives are administered to pregnant females, their presence in the body acts to inhibit the increase in oxytocin, oestrogen and PGF2a before labour, preventing uterine contraction, cervical dilation and expulsion of the foetus, resulting in foetal retention and death (JOHNSTON et al., 2001; LOPES, 2002).

After the foetuses die, their permanence in the uterine lumen can develop into foetal mummification or maceration (ALVES, 2012). Foetal mummification results from the incomplete resorption of retained foetuses, with bone structures remaining. This condition is associated with the integrity of the uterine sterile environment (SOUZA, 2012).

Foetal maceration occurs in the presence of pathogenic microorganisms that ascend from the vagina and find in retained foetuses a favourable environment for their installation and proliferation (JONES et al., 2000). The infectious process spreads, causing the uterus to be compromised or even ruptured. Subsequently, the microorganisms tend to invade neighbouring tissues, spreading throughout the body and thus developing septicaemia and toxemia (TONIOLLO and VICENTE, 2003).

Affected bitches may have purulent vaginal discharge with a foul odour, and residual tissue and bone may be found. In addition, the female shows signs of abdominal tenderness, anorexia, weight loss, fever, among other symptoms characteristic of sepsis, posing a great risk to the animal's life (BOLSON et al., 2004).

1.5.4. Breast tumour

Mammary tumours are predominantly hormone-dependent neoplasms characterised by the disorganised proliferation of mammary cells that start from genetic mutations (BOCARDO et al., 2008). These tumours account for approximately 52% of all neoplasms affecting female dogs. Of these, around 50% have malignant characteristics (QUEIROGA and LOPES, 2002).

Its aetiology may be related to hormonal, nutritional, genetic and environmental factors, the most important of which are age and prolonged exposure to hormones (SORENMO et al., 2011).

According to Fonseca and Daleck (2000), oestrogen and progesterone are substantial for the growth of mammary tumours and the process of carcinogenesis. Breast tissue, whether under normal or pathological conditions, contains a high concentration of specific receptors for these two hormones, thus revealing their hormonal dependence (LANA et al., 2007).

However, in cases of malignant neoplasms, the receptors for these hormones may be diminished or even non-existent, associated with a decrease in cell differentiation and progression of malignancy, representing a poor prognosis (FOSENCA and DALECK, 2000).

By binding to their receptors, oestrogens trigger proliferative activity in the breast epithelium, which increases the likelihood of genetic errors with oncogenic potential occurring. On the other hand, progesterone stimulates the production of growth hormone, which acts by inducing growth factors in the breast tissue, promoting its proliferation regardless of the presence or absence of neoplastic cells, thus leading to tumour development (FELICIANO et al., 2008).

Progestogen contraceptives act as described above, but because of their prolonged activity, they considerably increase the possibility of developing these breast neoplasms (MISDROP, 2002).

These tumours appear as nodules of varying size, adhered or not, single or multiple, and in some cases they have skin ulcerations or a well-established inflammatory process (SORENMO et al., 2011).

When malignant tumours form, their tumour cells can easily spread through the lymphatic and blood systems of the affected glands. As a consequence, regional metastases can form, affecting healthy breasts and other lymph nodes in the mammary chain, or distant metastases, attacking organs and systems, especially the lungs, liver and kidneys, resulting in their tissue destruction and altering their physiology (LANA et al., 2007).

Breast tumour treatment involves surgically removing the affected breast or, when necessary, the entire breast chain, as well as the lymph nodes associated with its drainage, to prevent recurrences or its spread to other regions (CASSALI et al., 2017).

CHAPTER 3

MATERIAL AND METHODS

3.1. Place of study

This study was carried out at the "Francisco Edilberto Uchoa Lopes" University Veterinary Hospital of the State University of Maranhão (UEMA), in São Luís - MA, by analysing the cases that occurred between January and December 2016.

3.2. Analysing medical records

The clinical records of all the female dogs seen at the HVU - UEMA in 2016 were analysed to identify which of them matched the profile proposed by this study, i.e. bitches affected by pyometra.

Among the patients with the condition described above, age, race and history of contraceptive use were analysed in order to assess whether these variables influenced the development of the disease.

3.3. Statistical Analysis

The statistical analysis was non-parametric, where the data was tabulated in Excel and then analysed.

CHAPTER 4

RESULTS AND DISCUSSION

In 2016, 2,325 female dogs were treated at the University Veterinary Hospital - UEMA in the municipality of São Luís. Of these, 271 were found to have the following pathologies: pyometra (4.81%), retained and dead foetuses (2.23%) and mammary tumours (4.6%) (figure 5).

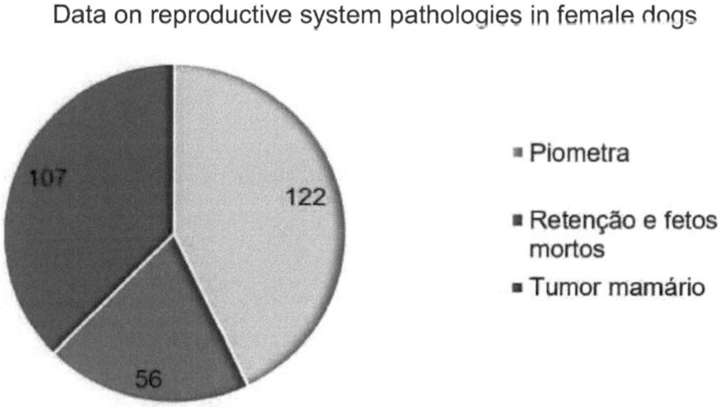

Data on reproductive system pathologies in female dogs

107
122
56
Piometra
Retenção e fetos mortos
Tumor mamário

Figure 3: Number of cases of pyometra, retained and dead foetuses and mammary tumours treated at the HVU - UEMA in 2016.
(Source: own authorship).

The use of contraceptives was employed by 98 bitches, while 106 did not and 67 did not have this information on their records. These figures show that 36.16% of owners (Figure 6) administer contraceptive drugs in an attempt to maintain reproductive control of their pets. This may be related to the easy commercial accessibility and low cost of these drugs (MONTANHA et al., 2012). This result was similar to that found in other studies, such as that by Dalla Nora and Freitas (2017), in which pyometra was more common than the other conditions (dead foetuses and mammary tumours), and studies by Sbiacheski and Da

Cruz (2016), who also reported a higher incidence of pyometra compared to the other alterations mentioned above.

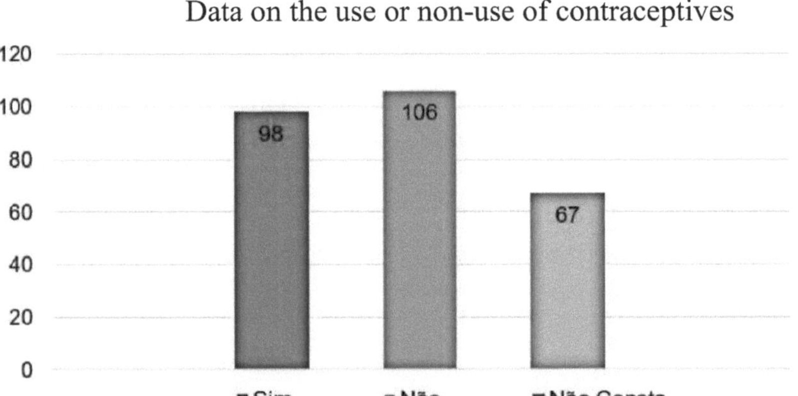

Figure 4: Number of cases of reproductive disorders related to the use or non-use of contraceptives. (Source: author)

The canine breeds most affected by pyometra were Sem Raça Definida (SRD), with 80 cases (71.43%), followed by Poodle, with 21 cases (18.75%) and the remaining 9.82% were distributed among the other breeds shown in Figure 7. In other studies, Coggan (2005) found SRDs and Poodles to be the most affected by pyometra, as shown in this study. Gorricho and Campos (2006) obtained similar results, finding a higher number of cases in SRD bitches and for the Yorkshire, Fox Paulistinha and Pinscher breeds. This reaffirms that there is no racial predisposition to this condition, as proposed by Murakami et al. (2011), since this disease has a greater hormonal than genetic influence.

Number of cases per breed diagnosed with pyometra

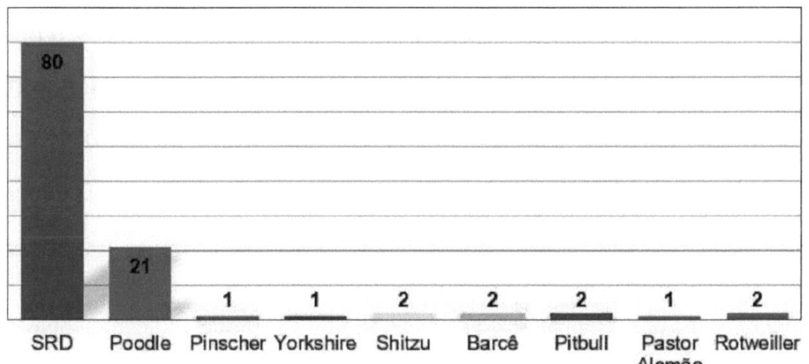

Figure 5: Dog breeds diagnosed with pyometra at the HVU - UEMA. (Source: author).

Of the 112 cases of pyometra diagnosed, 55 had used contraceptive drugs (49.10%), 44 had not (39.2%) and 13 (11.6%) did not have this information in their clinical records. These data corroborate the study carried out by Honório et al. (2017), where the number of cases of pyometra was also higher among bitches that used contraceptives. Chen et al. (2007) and Oliveira et al. (2008) also found that the origin of this pathology may be related to the administration of contraceptives.

In terms of age, pyometra occurred in 4.46% (5) of bitches under 1 year old, 33.92% (38) between 1 and 2 years old, 35.71% (40) between 3 and 6 years old and 25% (28) aged 7 years or more. The remaining 2.67% of cases were animals whose age was not stated in the clinical records. Thus, this condition was predominantly found in adult animals aged between 3 and 6 years (Table 1). Souza et al. (2014) showed that the age group between 3 and 5 years was more susceptible to developing this disease. Martins (2007) showed that the number of cases was higher in the 6-9 age group. It is known that the development of this pathology is related to the long exposure of the uterus to progesterone, which explains the higher incidence of pyometra in the 3 to 6 year old age group, followed by the 1 to 2 year old age group, since they have suffered greater exposure to contraceptives. This work corroborates the study by Evangelista et al. (2011) which concluded that young animals that use contraceptives become more susceptible to developing pyometra, although it is more common in adult and elderly animals.

Table 1. Number of cases of bitches affected by pyometra by age group and contraceptive use or not.

Age group (years)	Contraceptive use			
	Yes	**No**	**Not available**	**TOTAL**
< 1	2	2		4
1 - 2	18	16	4	38
3 - 6	20	13	7	40
7 - 10	14	12	2	28
Not available	1	1		2
TOTAL	55	44	13	112

CHAPTER 5

CONCLUSION

This study presented results relating to the use of contraceptives and the relationship with reproductive pathology influenced by their activity in the body, as well as age and breed. Adult female dogs aged between 3 and 6 years were more susceptible to pyometra, and there was no racial predisposition in any of the diseases studied.

The indiscriminate use of contraceptive drugs was common among animals affected by the aforementioned pathology. This demonstrates the importance of making owners aware of the danger that the use of these drugs poses to the health and well-being of pets. It is therefore essential that veterinarians keep owners informed about the risks and recommend surgical sterilisation as the safest control measure to avoid unwanted pregnancies.

CHAPTER 6

BIBLIOGRAPHICAL REFERENCES

ALLEN, W. E. Fertility and obstetrics in dogs. São Paulo: **Varela**, 197p. 1995.

ALVES, F. S. Extrauterine foetal mummification in a female dog - case report. **Clínica Veterinária**, v. 96, p. 88-94, 2012.

ANDRADE, S. F. Manual de Terapêutica Veterinária. 2ª ed. São Paulo: **Roca**, 2002.

ARAÚJO, E. K. D., et al. Main pathologies related to the adverse effects of the use of contraceptive drugs in cats. **PUBVET**, v. 11, p. 207-312, 2016.

ARNOLD, S.; HUBLER, M.; REICHLER, I. Canine pyometra: new approaches to an old disease. In: **World small veterinary Congress**. 2006.

BERNSTEIN, L.; ROSS, R. K. Endogenous hormones and breast cancer risk. **Epidemiologic reviews**, v. 15, n. 1, p. 48-65, 1993.

BOCARDO, M. et al. Hormonal influence on mammary carcinogenesis in bitches. **Rev. Ci. Med. Vet**, v. 6, n. 11, p. 1-6, 2008.

BOLSON, J. et al. Physometra in a female dog (Canis familiaris Linnaeus,

1758)-case report. **Arquivos de Ciências Veterinárias e Zoologia da UNIPAR**, v. 7, n. 2, p. 171-174, 2004.

CASSALI, G. D. et al. Consensus for the diagnosis, prognosis and treatment of canine mammary tumours. **Brazilian journal of veterinary pathology**, v. 4, n. 2, p. 153-180, 2017.

CHEN, R. F. F., ADDEO, P. M. D., SASAKI, A. Y. Open pyometra in a 10-month-old female dog. **Academic Journal: Animal Science**, v. 5, n. 3, 2017.

CHRISTIANSEN, I. B. J. Reproduction in dogs and cats. 1 ed. São Paulo: **Manole**, 1988.

COGGAN, J. A. **Microbiological study of intrauterine content and histopathology of the uterus of bitches with pyometra and research into virulence factors in E. coli strains and the potential risk to human health**. Doctoral thesis. University of São Paulo. 2005.

COLVILLE, T. P. Clinical anatomy and physiology for veterinary medicine. 2 ed. Rio de Janeiro: **Elsevier**, 2010.

CONCANNON, P. W. et al. Postimplantation increase in plasma fibrinogen concentration with increase in relaxin concentration in pregnant dogs. **American journal of veterinary research**, v. 57, n. 9, p. 1382-1385, 1996.

CONCANNON, P. W., MCCANN, J. P., TEMPLE, M. Biology and endocrinology of ovulation, pregnancy and parturition in the dog. **Journal of reproduction and fertility. Supplement**, v. 39, p. 325, 1989.

CONCANNON, P. W., VERSTEGEN, J. Some unique aspects of canine and feline female reproduction important in veterinary practice. In: **Proc.: 3rd World Congress of the World Small Anim. Vet. Assoc. 11-14 May 2005. Mexico City, Mexico**. 2005.

CONCANNON, P., TSUTSUI, T., SHILLE, V. Embryo development, hormonal requirements and maternal responses during canine pregnancy. **Journal of reproduction and fertility**. Supplement, v. 57, p. 169-179, 2001.

CRAIG, C. R. Modern Pharmacology. 4 ed. Rio de Janeiro: **Guanabara Koogan**, 1996.

CRIVELENLLENTI, L. Z., CRIVELENLLENTI S. B. Routine Cases in Small Animal Veterinary Medicine. São Paulo: **MedVet**, 2012.

DALLA NORA, L. R., DE FREITAS, E. S. Retrospective study of the pathological implications in female dogs exposed to contraceptive hormones from 2015 to 2017 in a veterinary clinic in the municipality of capitão leônidas marques/pr. In: Proceedings **of the National Congress of Veterinary Medicine FAG**. 2017.

DE CAMPOS, A. G., GORRICHO, C. M. Occurrence of pyometra in female dogs treated at veterinary clinics in the municipality of ituverava/sp in the first half of 2011. **Revista científica eletrônica de Medicina Veterinária**: Ano IX, n.18, São Paulo, 2012.

HONÓRIO, T. G. A. F. et al. Pathological implications after contraceptive use in female dogs located in Teresina-PI. **PUBVET**, v. 11, p. 103-206, 2016.

DE SOUZA, J. P. M. et al. Use of hormonal contraceptives and haematological status in the incidence of canine pyometra. **Veterinária e Zootecnia**, v. 21, n. 2, p. 275-278, 2014.

DELOUIS, C., RICHARD, P. La lactation La reproduction chez les mammifères et l'homme. p 487-514. **INRA-Ellipse, Paris, France,** 1991.

DERUSSI, A. A. P., LOPES, M. D. Physiology of ovulation, fertilisation and early embryonic development in the bitch. **Revista Brasileira de Reprodução Animal**, v. 33, n. 4, p. 231-237, 2009.

DUKES, H. H. Physiology of domestic animals. 11 ed. Rio de Janeiro: **Guanabara Koogan**, 1996.

DYCE, K. M.; SACK, W. O.; WENSING, C. J. G. Tratado de Anatomia Veterinária. 2. ed. Rio de Janeiro: **Guanabara Koogan**, 1997.

EILTS, B. E. et al. Factors affecting gestation duration in the bitch. **Theriogenology**, v. 64, n. 2, p. 242-251,2005.

ELLENPORT, C. R. General urogenital apparatus. In: GETTY, R. Anatomy of domestic animals. 5 ed. Rio de Janeiro: **Guanabara Koogan**, p.139. 1986.

ENGLAND, G.C.W. Pharnacological control of reproduction in the dog and bitch. In: SIMPSON, G.; ENGLAND, G.; HARVEY, M. Manual of small animal reproduction and neomatology. London: **BSVA**, p. 197122, 1998.

EPPIG J. J. **Oocyte control of ovarian follicular development and function in mammals**. Reproduction, v. 122, p. 829-838, 2001.

ETTINGER, S. J. Treatise on veterinary internal medicine. 3.ed. São Paulo: **Manole**, v.4, p.1857-1869. 1992.

EVANGELISTA, L. S. M. et al. Clinical and laboratory profile of female cats with pyometra before and after ovarian-hysterectomy. **Revista Brasileira de Reprodução Animal**, v. 35, n. 3, p. 347-351, 2011.

EVANS, Howard E.; DELAHUNTA, Alexander. Guide to the dissection of the dog. Rio de Janeiro: **Guanabara Koogan**, 2001.

FEITOSA, F. L. F. Veterinary semiology: the art of diagnosis. 3ed. São Paulo: **Roca**, 2014.

FELDMAN, E. C.; NELSON, R. W. Canine and feline endocrinology and reproduction. 3. ed. Philadelphia: **Williams & Wilkins**, 1344 p. 2003.

FELICIANO, M.A.R. et al. Mammary neoplasia in female dogs - literature review. **Electronic Scientific Journal of Veterinary Medicine**: Year IX, n.1, São Paulo, 2012.

FERREIRA P.C.C. **Evaluation of haemodiafiltration in the perioperative period of ovarian-salpingo-hysterectomy in bitches with pyometra refractory to conservative treatment of acute renal failure**. PhD thesis, University of São Paulo, São Paulo. 2006.

FERREIRA, C. R., LOPES, M. D. Complex endometrial cystic hyperplasia/piometra in bitches - review. **Revista Clínica Veterinária**, n.25, p.36-44, 2000.

FILGUEIRA, K. D., REIS, P. F. C. C., PAULA, V. V. Feline mammary hyperplasia: therapeutic success with the use of aglepristone. **Ciência Animal Brasileira**, v. 9, n. 4 p. 1010-1016, 2008.

FINGLAND, R. B. Ovariohysterectomy. **BOJRAB, MJ Current techniques in small animal surgery**, v. 3, p. 375-381, 1996.

FONSECA, C.S.; DALECK, C.R. Mammary neoplasms in bitches: hormonal influence and effects of ovariohysterectomy as adjuvant therapy. **Ciência Rural**, v.30, n.4, p.731-735, 2000.

FOSSUM, T. W. Small animal surgery. In: HEDLUND, C. S. Surgery of the reproductive and genital systems. 3. ed. Rio de Janeiro: **Elsevier**, p. 28;731. 2008.

FOSTER, R. A. Reproductive system of the female. MCGAVIN, MD,

ZACHARY, JF Bases of Veterinary Pathology. 4. ed. Rio de Janeiro: **Elsevier**, p. 1263-1315, 2009.

GETTY, R. Sisson and Grossman's anatomy of domestic animals. 5 ed. Rio de Janeiro: **Guanabara Koogan**, 1986.

GREGERSON, K. A. Prolactin: structure, function, and regulation of secretion. In: Neill, J.D. (Ed) Knobil **and Neill's physiology of** reproduction. 3 ed. v.1. Sant Louis: **Elsevier Academic Press**, p. 1703-1726, 2006.

HAFEZ, B., HAFEZ, E. S. E. Animal reproduction. 7. ed. São Paulo: **Manole**, 2004.

HAGMAN, R., KINDAHL, H., LAGERSTEDT, A.-S. Pyometra in bitches induces elevated plasma endotoxin and prostaglandin F 2a metabolite levels. **Acta Veterinaria Scandinavica**, v. 47, n. 1, p. 55, 2006.

HARDY, R. M., OSBORNE, C. A. Canine pyometra: pathophysiology, diagnosis and treatment of uterine and extra-uterine lesions. Journal of the America **Animal Hospital Association**, v. 10, p. 245-267, 1974.

HEDLUND, C. S. et al. Surgery of the reproductive and genital systems. **FOSSUM, TW Small Animal Surgery**, v. 2, p. 619672, 2002.

HOFFMANN, B. et al. Ovarian and pituitary function in dogs after hysterectomy. **Journal of reproduction and fertility**, v. 96, n. 2, p. 837-

845, 1992.
HOLST, P. A., PHEMISTER, R. D. Temporal sequence of events in the estrous cycle of the bitch. **American journal of veterinary research**, v. 36, n. 5, p. 705-706, 1975.

JEFFCOATE, I. A.; LINDSAY, F. E. Ovulation detection and timing of insemination based on hormone concentrations, vaginal cytology and the endoscopic appearance of the vagina in domestic bitches. **Journal of reproduction and fertility. Supplement**. v. 39, p. 277-287, 1989.

JOHNSTON, S. D. Pseudopregnancy in the bitch. **Current Veterinary Theriogenology. 2nd ed. Philadelphia: W. B. Saunders Co**, p. 490-491, 1986.

JONES, T. C.; HUNT, R. D.; KING, N. W. Veterinary Pathology. 6.ed. São Paulo: **Manole**, p. 1200, 2000.

JUNQUEIRA, L. C.; CARNEIRO, J. Female reproductive system. **Histologia Básica Ed**, v. 10, p. 449-452, 2004.

KATZUNG, B. G. Basic and Clinical Pharmacology. 8 ed. Rio de Janeiro: **Guanabara Koogan**, 2003.

KONIG, H. E.; LIEBICH, H. G. Female genital organs. Anatomy of Domestic Animals. Porto Alegre: **Artmed**, 2004.

LADD, A. et al. Development of an antifertility vaccine for pets based on active immunisation against luteinizing hormone-releasing hormone. **Biology of Reproduction**, v. 51, n. 6, p. 1076-1083, 1994.

LIMA, J. G. P. et al. **Contraceptive use in female dogs**: problem or solution? 2009.

LINDE-FORSBERG, C., ENEROTH, A. Abnormalities in pregnancy, parturition, and the periparturient period. **Textbook of veterinary internal medicine**, v. 7, p. 1890-1901,2005.

LOPES, M. D. Hormone Therapy in Small Animals. In: Paulista Congress of Small Animal Veterinary Clinicians. Proceedings. São Paulo: **National Association of Small Animal Veterinary Clinicians of São Paulo**, 2002.

LUZ, M. R. Childbirth in turkeys and cats. **Canine and feline reproduction topics by authors**, 2004.

LUZ, M. R., FREITAS, P. M. C., PEREIRA, E. Z. Pregnancy and labour in bitches: physiology, diagnosis of pregnancy and treatment of dystocia. **Revista Brasileira de Reprodução Animal**, v. 29, n. 3/4, p. 142-150, 2005.

MADDISON, J. E., PAGE, S., CHURCH, D. Small animal clinical pharmacology. Rio de Janeiro: **Elsevier**, 2010.

MARTINS, D. G. Cystic endometrial hyperplasia/pyometra complex: pathophysiology, clinical and laboratory characteristics and therapeutic approach. **Jaboticabal. Unesp- Jaboticabal**, 2007.

MARTINS, D.G. **Cystic Endometrial Hyperplasia/Piometra Complex in** MIGLINO, M. A. et al. The carnivore pregnancy: the development of the embryo and foetal membranes. **Theriogenology**, v. 66, n. 6, p. 1699-1702, 2006.

MISDROP, W. Tumours of the mammary gland. In: MEUTEN, D. J. Tumors in domestic animals. 4. ed. Iowa: **Blackwell Publishing**, p. 575-606. 2002.

MONTANHA, F. P.; CORRÊA, C. S. S.; PARRA, T. C. Foetal maceration in a cat due to the use of contraceptives - case report. **Revista Científica Eletrônica de Medicina Veterinária**, v. 10, n. 9, p. 1- 6, 2012.

MUNNICH, Andrea; KUCHENMEISTER, Uwe. Dystocia in Numbers-Evidence-Based Parameters for Intervention in the Dog: Causes for Dystocia and Treatment Recommendations. **Reproduction in domestic animals**, v. 44, n. s2, p. 141-147, 2009.

MURAKAMI, V. Y. et al. Pyometra - case report. **Electronic Scientific Journal of Veterinary Medicine**. Year IX, n. 17, São Paulo, 2011. NELSON, R. W., COUTO, C. G. Disorders of the vagina and uterus. In: Fundamentals of small animal internal medicine. Rio de Janeiro: **Guanabara Koogan**, p. 486-87, 2006.

OLIVEIRA, N. G. et al. Use of aglepristone and cloprostenol in the treatment of pyometra in a female dog - case report. 2007.

PEREIRA, C. P. et al. Comparative anatomical study of mammary lymphatic vascularisation in healthy and neoplasm-affected bitches. **Brazilian Journal of Morphology Science**, v. 17, n. 490, p. 135, 2000.

PRETZER, S. D. Clinical presentation of canine pyometra and mucometra: A review, **Theriogenology**, v. 70, p. 359-363, 2008.

PREVIATO, P. F. G. et al. Morphological changes in the genital organs of dogs and cats from rural villages in the region of Umuarama, PR. **Arquivos de Ciências Veterinárias e Zoologia da UNIPAR**, v. 8, n. 2, p. 105-110, 2005.

SBIACHESKI, D. T., DA CRUZ, F. S. F. Use of progestogens and their adverse effects in small animals. **Salon of Knowledge**, v. 2, n. 2, 2016.

SCHIOCHET, F. et al. Laparoscopic ovariohysterectomy in a cat with mummified foetuses - case report. **Revista portuguesa de ciências veterinária**, v. 102, p. 361-364, 2007.

SLATTER. D. Manual of Small Animal Surgery. 2 vols. 3ed. São Paulo: **Manole**, 2007.

SMITH F.O. Canine pyometra. **Theriogenology**. v. 66, p. 610-2, 2006.

SORENMO, K. U. et al. Development, anatomy, histology, lymphatic drainage, clinical features, and cell differentiation markers of canine mammary gland neoplasms. **Veterinary pathology**, v. 48, n. 1, p. 8597, 2011.

SOUZA, M. R. et al. Stillbirth and foetal mummification in pigs. **Revista Eletrônica Nutritime**, a. 163, v. 9, n° 03 p.1787- 1800. 2012.

STEPHEN, J. B., SHERDING, R. G. Saunders Manual - Small Animal Clinic. 3ª ed. São Paulo: **Roca,** 2008.

SUGIURA, K. et al. Effect of ovarian hormones on periodic changes in immune resistance associated with estrous cycle in the beagle bitch. **Immunobiology**, v. 209, n. 8, p. 619-627, 2004.

THATCHER, W. W.; MEYER, M. D.; DANET-DESNOYERS, G. Maternal recognition of pregnancy. **Journal of reproduction and fertility**, v. 49, p. 15-28, 1995.

TONIOLO, G. H., VICENTE, W. R. R. Manual of Veterinary Obstetrics. São Paulo: **Varela**, 2003.

TYLER, J. Clinical examination of the mammary glands. In: **Radostits, O. M., Mayhew, I. G. J., Houston, D. M., Clinical examination and diagnosis in veterinary medicine, Rio de Janeiro: Guanabara Koogan**, p. 572-578, 2002.

VERSTEGEN, J.; DHALIWAL, G.; VERSTEGEN-ONCLIN, K. Mucometra, cystic endometrial hyperplasia, and pyometra in the bitch: Advances in treatment and assessment of future reproductive success, **Theriogenology**, v. 70, p. 364-374, 2008.

VIGO, F., LUBIANCA, J. N., CORLETA, H. E. Progestogens: pharmacology and clinical use - Review. **FEMINA**, v. 39, n. 3, 2011.

WEILENMANN, R. et al. Estradiol and progesterone concentrations in the plasma of nonpregnant bitches during the sexual cycle. **Schweizer Archiv fur Tierheilkunde**, v. 135, n. 2, p. 51-57, 1993.

ZUCCARI, D. A. P. C., SANTANA, A. E., ROCHA, N. S. Expression of intermediate filaments in the diagnosis of mammary tumours in bitches. **Arquivo Brasileiro de Medicina Veterinária e Zootecnia**, v.54, n.6, 2002.

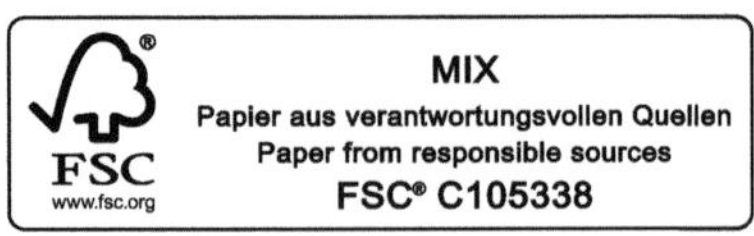

Printed by Books on Demand GmbH, Norderstedt / Germany